Cancer
Winning the Battle

How To Prepare Your Body – Not Only To Fight But To Win

Cathy Ostema

Introduction

Cancer is a horrible disease. It effects millions of people, including their friends and families.

This book is about getting healthy. It's about being healthy to the point that your body can work the way it was meant to work. And that means allowing it to fight and beat cancer.

This book is also about getting healthy no matter what disease you have. It doesn't have to be cancer. It can be that you have some other disease or simply want to get a little healthier so you're around to enjoy your grandchildren (when you're old enough).

Follow the steps included in this book and you will see your life improve. These are not hard steps. Most of them you probably are already aware of. But I find without support to remind and push us, we tend to forget these steps.

The human body is designed to beat disease. You can do it ! I'll help you.

Chapter 1

In today's world, with its fast food, radiation-producing technology, and GMOs swimming among and mixing in with a thousand other pollutants, it's no wonder cancer is on the rise.

We're told a food is good for us, and then a couple of months later, we're told it's cancer-causing.

The FDA passes chemicals without testing them. And, of course, big business is paying behind closed doors to ensure this happens. So we ingest products we believe are safe, only to find out a few years later that they cause numerous diseases.

Then you travel down the road a few years, and you find yourself walking out of the doctor's office shaking in fear because they found a "lump." You swear you eat right; you exercise; you pray. So how did this happen to you? More importantly, why?

When this happens, your world is turned upside down, and you don't know which way to turn.

The doctors are telling you that you need aggressive surgery, chemo, and/or radiation treatments. But you've heard horror stories about people that go through the treatments.

There must be another way!

I'm here to tell you, for many of you, there is. And it's not dangerous or expensive or hard to do. It doesn't cause health issues down the road like the treatments do.

Am I telling you to go against your doctor's advice? NO. I would never do that. You do what you feel is right for you. I am not suggesting you do anything different than what you and your doctor decide.

And I am not telling you that I can cure you. In fact, I don't think anyone can cure you, except you. You have the power inside of you to handle this issue; you just need help in figuring out how to unlock the secret steps to success.

What I am telling you is that it's good to have an open mind, do your research, check out your options. And make up your own mind. Don't blindly follow what I say, and don't blindly follow what your doctor says. I'm telling you to make informed decisions. Use your heart and your mind both. Listen to your gut, and do what is right for you.

In the following chapters, you'll learn how to make changes in your life that I believe can improve your life in wonderful ways. Even if you don't have cancer, if you follow the recommendations you find in this book, your health will very likely improve. You'll have more energy, feel better, lose weight, balance your mood, feel stronger, and be happier. It's worth it for you to settle in and be determined to do everything you can to live the best life you can. So read on, and may the universe respond exactly how you dream it will.

Chapter 2

I offer my clients a Healthy Body Program, where I take people through twelve weeks of one-on-one sessions to prepare their body to fight cancer or any other disease. But I want to reach more people. This is too important not to share. So, what I've done is condensed the information from my twelve-week program to fit into this book. I have not included any of the important bonus calls or free gifts that come with the program. I left out the recipes and handouts. And you aren't getting the entire program or the one-on-one attention. But you are getting enough information to get you started on the right path to a new, healthy you.

You can contact me at 616-204-8585 for more information.

Happy reading and healthy life to you!

Chapter 3

Let's start by answering the question, *what is cancer?* What is happening in the body that allows the cells to mutate?

The quick explanation starts with your genes.

Our genes determine who we are, what we look like, and how long we live. And in return, what you eat, think, believe, do, breathe, drink, and feel determines what your genes are doing. So, in other words, A (genes) equals B (your actions) equals A equals B and on and on.

We have the ability to change our gene expression, and we do this on a daily basis. In fact, we do this on a moment-to-moment basis, switching on and off genes throughout the day.

There are little tags that attach to your genes called epigenomes. These little tags "turn on" or "turn off" your genes. We all have methyl tags, which turn genes off, and acetyl tags, which turn genes on. Epigenomes make decisions on what our cells should be or how they should act.

So...

Histone acetylation activates your genes or turns them on.

DNA methylation quiets the genes or turns them off.

When a person gets cancer, it means that the genes that prevent cell overgrowth have been turned off.

The way to prevent or reverse this is by turning on and off the correct genes.

And the way we do this is by the foods we eat, meditations, and exercise.

One of the ways to help your genes get back in proper order is by re lieving stress in the mind and body. This is one of the most important keys to guiding our genes in the direction of healing that we want them to go in. Another way is exercise, like yoga, which has been proven to reduce oxidative stress. Yet another is with our diet, by eating foods rich in antioxidants to fight oxidants in the body. One great food to try is green tea, since it has a type of antioxidant that can help prevent cancer.

We live in a world that is filled with toxins; sadly, most of these are manmade. The World Wildlife Fund (WWF) ran tests on some forty-seven members of the European Parliament. They found that, on average, per member, there were 41 synthetic chemicals in the blood. Another report found 350 contaminants in breast milk. These contaminants included DDT, dioxins, and flame retardant.

As I wrote above, diet is important. The foods you eat can change your epigenomes, or the switches on your genes. Examples of this are the nutrients sulforaphane, which is found in broccoli, and diallyl disulfide (DADS), which is found in garlic. Both of these substances increase histone acetylation in the body and turn on the anti-cancer genes. What we eat has a huge impact on our health, right down to our genes. So if you're turning on your anti-cancer genes, you are turning on your fighters. You are priming your body to fight the invader cells.

You hold the power to change who you are and how your body reacts to disease.

You are in control.

Chapter 4

So, now the question is, how do you go about making changes? The easiest way is to have a mentor or someone who is willing to hold you accountable. You didn't set out to get sick. And you may or may not know what you need to change. But having someone to back you up helps you figure out the changes that you need to make and helps you actually stick to them. It takes sixty-six days to make a behavior a habit. There is an old myth that it takes twenty-one days, but that has been proven to be incorrect.Sixty-six days, a little over two months, is the actual length of time it takes to make something a habit.

That's all it takes to change your world and become a healthier person. But you must make the changes. They won't happen on their own. You can't read this book and be healthy simply because you read it. You have to follow the suggestions and do the work.

Making one or two changes every week is all it takes. I would advise against attempting to make all the changes at once. I believe that doing so would be a shock to your system. If you've been living in a fast food world, smoking, eating junk food, and being sedentary and stressed out, and you try to change your entire diet and lifestyle all at once, your ability to be successful at maintaining those changes are slim.

Be patient with yourself. That doesn't mean slacking and not implementing the suggestions. It means that, if you slip on a section, you shouldn't stress out about it. When you become aware that you have slipped up, stop, take a deep breath, exhale, remind yourself why you're doing this and how much better you're going to feel, and start over. Start over right then and there—not the next day. Do it right then, in the moment.

Life is about choices; you have the choice to make changes. That option to make a choice is happening at every moment of every day. You can start over every single moment. We live in a marvelous world where we have freewill, and you have the power to use that freewill. I'm here to encourage you to do just that.

Imagine what you want your life to look like in six months from now. How is it different from your life now? Write down exactly what you want your life to be like. Use your imagination. There are no rules here; this is your life. You can make it any life you want. There is no right or wrong. You don't have to tell or show anyone what you write. Free your inhibitions and make it the best life you can possibly imagine. What do you want in your relationships or job? Where do you live? What does your home look like? Who is in your social circle or who do you want to be with? What do you want to experience, do, or try? What is your spiritual life like? How do you look and feel physically? Who have you become?

Write it all down; don't skip any of it. Create your world. Take your time and think this through. Remember, this is your life you're writing down—make it fabulous.

Now read it to yourself and visualize that life. How does it feel in your mind to have that life? Are you happy, healthy, and excited about life? Do you have a purpose in life?

Now your job is to create that life you dreamed about.

This is now one of your goals. We should always have short-term goals and long-term goals. This is a long-term goal. Now we need to start making changes to create that life. A way to start that is to take hold of your health and be the boss.

Chapter 5

Okay, so now you've figured out who you want to be, but you need to know how to go about becoming that person. Let's start with some changes that you can make.

First of all, how and what should you eat? How much of each food group do you need? What are these magic foods that can turn on and off genes?

Let's start with the amounts of carbs, protein, and fats you need daily. The percentages in which each group should be eaten differ with age, but for this book, we are using the percentages for adults.

The diet of adults should be made up of about 45-65 percent carbs. These are healthy carbs, not a white bun from a fast food joint or a cookie that stared you in the face until you ate it. We are talking about carbs that you get from vegetables, fruits, and legumes.

Protein should make up about 10-35 percent. This would include legumes and organic, free-range, GMO free, antibiotic- and hormone free, pasture-raised meat. I know that's a lot of details, but they are important details.

And about 20-35 percent of your food intake should be healthy fat. Healthy fats include avocado, coconut oil, olive oil (on salads, not to cook with), olives, nuts, and seeds.

Breaking that down even further, for optimal health, you should have raw veggies, cooked veggies, nuts, and/or seeds at every meal. Most cooked veggies lose a lot of their micronutrients, which are needed by the body to stay strong, in the cooking process, so you want some of your veggies raw. This can mean eating a simple salad or a more complex raw food dish.

Also, by cooking foods at high temperatures, we create byproducts called acrylamide and thermolyzed casein. These have been linked to cancer. This means that, when you do cook food, it is best to use a lower setting on the burner and cook your food slower.

Humans, like other animals, need what is called "sun energy." This is available only in raw food or directly from the sun, through the skin. When you consume raw foods, your body stores the "sun energy" as "biophotons."

What's really interesting is that our bodies emit biophotons as a means of communication between cells. We also emit biophotons out of our body. The higher our stress and/or the free radicals in our body, the higher the output of biophotons we emit. Since we need these biophotons to allow our cells to communicate, we can't afford to be under a lot of unnecessary stress. Meditation can slow this process down. When we meditate, we allow our "monkey minds" to quiet down. Our society has us running in circles. We are thinking constantly. And, often, we are thinking about our daily worries, things that are piling up on us. We worry about getting chores done, money, family, social status, health, work issues, and more. A lot of people have worries stacking up on them to the point where they end up taking medication to control their worries.

And, of course, medication often leads us to more health issues down the road.

Meditation, on the other hand, is freeing. It is calming and gentle. There are no ill side effects. And instead of generating health issues like medications can, it actually helps turn your genes back to where they belong.

When we meditate, we let go of worry and allow our minds to be still. Our bodies increase our immune system, we have less anxiety, we increase our focus and memory, our blood pressure is reduced, our heart and brain issues are lessened, and inflammation is reduced. On top of all that, meditation also helps improve your mood and allows for more creativity. AND it helps slow the release of biophotons.

Biophotons hold bio-information. This information helps order and regulate your vital processes. We need biophotons. Meditation slows their release, and eating raw food is one of the best and easiest ways to add them to our system. The other best way is to spend time in the sun. That is also a healthy way to get your vitamin D. (But for many of us who live in the Northern states, it isn't possible to be out in the sunshine every day of the year.)

So we can meditate to feel relaxed, so we don't have an overabundance of biophotons released out of our bodies.

Eating Veggies

How many veggies do we need? That depends on where you live. If you live in Alaska, your body requires more fat and less veggies to stay healthy. If you live in Florida, your body will need more fruits and veggies and lower fats.

What I find works the best for most people is having one-third of your plate made up of raw veggies and one-third made up of cooked veggies (some veggies are better for you if slightly cooked). Add in 20-30 percent fat, such as avocado, coconut oil, olives, and organic, free-range, grass-fed butter, and include 10-30 percent protein and 45-65 percent healthy carbs.

"Carbs" does not mean a lot of bread. Remember that your veggies are carbs! Figuring this out for your plate is a lot easier than it sounds.

If one-third of your plate is a salad with avocado and maybe some nuts on top and/or a little olive oil, you probably just satisfied the raw food and fat percentages both. Maybe add a piece of fresh fruit, and you have it made. Now add one-third of your plate in cooked veggies; that's easy to do. Some slightly steamed broccoli fills the order. Or some butternut squash. Maybe you like sautéed brussels sprouts with lemon and onions. Whatever vegetable you like, cooked whatever way you like it, should, for the most part, be fine.

That leaves one third of your plate for protein and carbs to share. And you already have some carbs from the veggies on your plate.

All your veggies should be organic. Fresh is best, and frozen is second best. Please don't eat canned veggies. Most of the cans used for vegetables are coated with bisphenol A (BPA). This is to keep bacteria out of the can. It also prevents the metal from corroding. BPA is linked to endocrine disorders, heart disease and cancer and may alter neural development fetuses.

Canned vegetables are also generally extremely high in sodium and contain sulfites as a preservative. Some people are allergic to sulfites.

When we eat fresh vegetables, they carry more nutrients than canned. And if you buy local, you get a LOT more nutrient value. When we buy produce that has to travel for days to get to us, the produce has to be picked before it has ripened naturally on the plant. Otherwise it would be overripe by the time it reached us. It isn't really ripening on its travels; it's beginning the rotting process. The produce is losing nutrients as it rots.

So by the time it reaches the store, it has lost both flavor and nutritional value.

Buying local means you are buying a vegetable that was picked ripe from the plant and is full of flavor and nutrients. Especially if it is organic. When we purchase local, organic produce, we are getting all the flavor and nutrients. And what we are not getting is all the cancer-causing chemicals from the pesticides. Also, most people say organic has more flavor!

And, if you really want to kick start your health, then eat mostly cruciferous veggies and leafy greens. (Cruciferous veggies include, but are not limited to, arugula, bok choy, broccoli, brussels sprout, cabbage, cauliflower, collard greens, kale, and watercress.)

Cruciferous veggies are loaded with phytochemicals, great vitamins, and needed minerals. They contain healthy fiber. They also lower your risk for developing cancer by protecting your cells from DNA damage. Cruciferous veggies stop carcinogens from reacting. And, these powerhouses reduce oxygen-free radicals and have antiviral and antibacterial properties. They help stop the migration of tumor cells, help prevent tumor blood vessel formation, and have anti-inflammatory properties.

Leafy greens would include, but are not limited to romaine lettuce, leaf lettuce, kale, collard greens, swiss chard, and spinach. **Leafy greens** have **fiber**, **folate**, **flavonoids**, and **carotenoids**.

Fiber can help prevent colon cancer. Fiber adds bulk to your stools and moves them quickly through your intestines. This limits how long your body is in contact with toxins. Fiber with water can actually dilute toxins that are carcinogenic. It also encourages the growth of healthy bacteria and can lower the amount of unhealthy bacteria in your intestines.

Folate has been shown to help prevent several cancers and heart disease.

Flavonoids work as antioxidants in your body, and studies are now linking them to preventing several cancers.

Carotenoids also work in your body as an antioxidant and have been found to have strong cancer-fighting abilities. Carotenoids are converted into vitamin A in your body; although, some carotenoids are not able to be converted. Carotenoids have been found to have strong cancer-fighting abilities. Some foods with carotenoids include sweet potatoes, carrots, tomatoes, and dark leafy greens.

So you can see why adding a salad to your plate is a great idea. Leafy greens and bright-colored veggies are essential for a healthy body. What kind of veggies are you planning on eating tonight?

(Note: All vitamins, minerals, and fiber should be obtained from natural food sources. When taken in pill form, some can actually increase a person's risk of cancer.)

Fats

What are good fats, and what do they do for us?

For starters, healthy fats help us to feel full longer. They also are carriers for fat-soluble vitamins such as vitamins A, D, E, and K. They can take away the bad cholesterol from our system and raise the good cholesterol. This means you will have cleaner arteries or, in other words, less plaque build-up. The body gets energy from fat, gives our brain and nerves the ability to function properly, and helps us have healthy skin.

Healthy fats help you lose weight and help protect your internal organs! They can surround your organs and become a cushion of protection for sudden impacts or when organs are jostled around. This allows the organs to slide against each other rather than rub, stick, or tear.

Healthy fats include avocado; olives; olive oil (used in salads, not cooked with); coconut oil; salmon (wild caught); flax seed; nuts; seeds; and grass-fed, organic butter.

Fats should be included with every meal. It's easy to add them in. An avocado or coconut oil added to a smoothie is easy. And the avocado makes a smoothie creamy and thick. Olive oil added to a salad is quick. Nuts, seeds, flax seeds can be added to cooked veggies, a salad, or a smoothie. And, of course, salmon can be a main entree or used in a salad. Try adding a little to your next omelet. There is no reason to not get your healthy fats in.

Sweeteners

There is some controversy over whether sugar is harmful for those with cancer or not. Sugar feeds cancer. This is a true statement. And there is some evidence that high sugar consumption is linked to some cancers. What is also true is that sugar feeds ALL of your cells and you need *some*. If you consume too much, though, you risk becoming obese, and that, as well, increases your risk of developing cancer.

I used to suggest that people eliminate all sugar from their diet. But there is enough evidence to prove this to be unnecessary.

That does not mean to run out and eat white sugar! White sugar is never a healthy choice. It is a refined, highly processed substance that is no longer a food. There is no nutritional value to it. Additionally, brown sugar and the "raw sugar" that comes in the little brown packets are nothing more than white sugar with some of the molasses added back into it.

But there are a few sweeteners that are healthy and that have not been stripped of their vital nutrients as white sugar has been. These are fine to use in small amounts.

Healthy sugars include:

Maple syrup – Maple syrup has lots of minerals in it. It offers iron, calcium, zinc, manganese, and potassium. But don't use the maple syrup from the typical grocery store because it frequently has corn syrup added. Get pure maple syrup from a health food store to ensure you are getting a healthy, pure product.

Honey – Only buy raw, local honey. You want local honey because it is produced from the plants that grow in the area. This can help the system fight against allergies. Also, when you buy it raw, you know it doesn't have corn syrup added. In addition, honey has vitamin B-6 and vitamin C. And it has three times the value of riboflavin that maple syrup has.

Coconut sugar – Coconut sugar is another good sweetener that is fairly new and growing in popularity. Coconut sugar is made similarly to the way maple syrup is made, and it also retains some of its nutritional value. It is also a low glycemic food, meaning it won't raise your blood sugar levels quickly. It has a very nice flavor to it. I also have coconut sugar in my cupboards. I find that sometimes I feel like I have to use a little more of it than I do honey or maple syrup. So the one I use depends on what I'm doing.

Coconut sugar also has some good nutrient values. It is high in potassium and includes nitrogen, phosphorus, calcium, magnesium, sodium, chlorine, sulfur, and trace amounts of boron, zinc, manganese, iron, and copper. It also has six amino acids that help with overall growth and repair, hormones, and enzymes. It offers vitamin B-8 (also called inositol), which helps with healthy cell development. It also has thiamine, riboflavin, para-aminobenzoic acid, pyridoxal, pantothenic acid, nicotinic acid, biotin, folic acid, choline, and trace levels of vitamin B-12. The B vitamins are essential for proper metabolic function; healthy skin, muscles, and nervous and immune systems; and for aiding cell development.

Stevia – Stevia is also a good sweetener, but I find it can have an aftertaste that some people don't care for. I personally don't care for the taste, but a lot of people like it. I like using maple syrup, honey, or coconut sugar because they all have added nutritional value.

I'm not saying to eat a cup of any of these sweeteners in order to obtain your minerals or vitamins or on a daily basis. But if you are going to use a little sugar, I believe these to be healthier choices.

Proteins – The Safe List

All meat and eggs should be antibiotic-free, hormone-free, organic, free-range, pasture-raised, humanely-raised, and not fed soy.

Yes, that is a long list. The alternative is eating something that is full of chemicals and has been tortured and lived in fear and/or agony. Not only is that putting the wrong hormones in your body, but it means you are condoning that type of farming and supporting the people who would do that to other creatures. That is not good for them.

There are good, valid reasons for adding meat into your diet and also for being vegetarian or a vegan. The following is simple info if you are a meat eater. If you are a non-meat eater you can simple skip down to the section on gluten, unless you are interested in the information provided.

The following are a healthy choice if you are a meat eater:

· Chicken

· Fish

· Beans

· Eggs

The following are things you should avoid:

Red meat – includes beef, pork, and lamb. (And, yes, bacon is red meat.)

Red meat contains N-glycolylneuraminic acid (Neu5Gc). This is a sugar that is naturally found in red meat animals but is not naturally occurring in humans. When we consume this sugar, our bodies see it as a foreign substance and attack it. Your immune system turns on and sends out antibodies to combat it. This causes inflammation in the system. And inflammation can eventually lead to cancer.

Overeating protein is not healthy either. When the body consumes protein and we reach our needed limit, we have to eliminate the rest. Our systems are not capable of saving or storing the excess. So when we consume excessive amounts, especially from animal protein, we still have to eliminate the rest. Our kidneys and liver have to go into overtime to eliminate this excess protein, and this causes an overabundance of toxic byproducts. These toxins are then flushed out through the kidneys. The kidneys are put in a position where they are overworked, and you can develop kidney stones, bone loss, osteoporosis, damage to the kidneys, immune issues, and arthritis, as well as increase your risk of cancer and/or create low-energy. So, when you are eating meat, limit how much you consume. This is why one-third of your plate is for carbs and protein to share.

Eliminating red meat from your diet helps relieve this stress on your organs and lessens your chance of developing cancer due to toxic overload from excessive protein.

Wheat, Rye, Barley, and Sometimes Oats

Foods containing grains like wheat, rye, barley, and oats can cause several health problems, including cancer, because of several different components that are contained in it.

Let's start by talking about the one that you have probably already heard of: gluten.

I could write an entire book on gluten. Let me just say here that you want to avoid it. Gluten causes inflammation of the gut in over eighty percent of the population. Ninety-nine percent of the population is susceptible to developing antibodies against gluten. We are all basically gluten intolerant. It's just that we all have different thresholds for our point of disease.

Gluten is found in the grains wheat, rye, and barley. And, of course, it is found in any foods made with any of these grains. This includes the foods you would think of, such as cereal, bread, cakes, and pastries, but gluten is also found in foods you might not think of. Gluten is found in soy sauce, couscous, seitan, wheat bran, wheat germ, bulgur, barley malt, soups, pasta, beer, gravy, sauces, dressings, bouillon cubes, some candies, imitation fish and crab, some lunch meats and hot dogs, modified food starch, seasoned rice, and seasoned snack foods. No wonder it's such a problem!

Although oats are a gluten-free food, they are often listed as containing gluten because they are generally manufactured in factories that have gluten products or have been contaminated during the harvesting process and/or the planting process. The oats become contaminated with the gluten and can cause reactions in the consumer. Look for oats that are labeled "gluten free." Oats labeled gluten-free should be produced in a factory free of gluten grains.

If you feel like you have to have bread and bread products, there are healthy gluten-free recipes out there. I don't recommend store-bought gluten-free foods because of other ingredients that may be added to them.

It is also important to know that just because something is labeled as "wheat-free," it does not mean it is gluten-free. It means it is wheat-free. It may have barley or rye in it, so always check your labels.

So what makes gluten such a problem for people? Gluten contains a protein called gliadin. Gliadin is structured similarly to other proteins that are in our tissues and organs. Our bodies may make antibodies to attack the gliadin protein in our organs, such as the thyroid, and end up causing autoimmune disease like hypothyroidism.

Gluten affects our bodies in several different ways:

- **Inflammation** – The inflammatory effect of gluten in our gut causes our intestinal cells to die off earlier than they would otherwise. This causes leaky gut, which allows for bacteria and other toxins to travel between the gut and into the blood stream. This can end with your body having autoimmune attacks on itself. It also means that you are not getting all of the nutrients out of your food because it isn't digesting properly.

- **Heart disease** – If your body creates antibodies against gluten, you can end up with heart disease because these antibodies have been shown to attack the heart tissue.

- **Cancer** – Gluten has been shown to be cancer-promoting, if not actually cancer-causing. Either way, it is strongly linked to cancer.

The second problem that we have with wheat is wheat germ agglutinin (WGA), which is a "lectin problem." This is found in wheat and may be linked to a lot of the health issues caused by wheat. The problem with lectin is that it is found in all grains, seeds, legumes, tomatoes, potatoes, and dairy. And it has the potential to lower our quality of life and even how long we live.

WGA lectins are hardy and tough. They are small and hard to breakdown. And they accumulate in bodily tissues where they intermingle with normal tissue and upset the normal functions.

WGA lectin is so strong and resistant that scientists have used it as an insecticide in GMO plants. And then we eat these plants, thus consuming even more WGA lectin than used to be present in wheat.

One way to see the increase of issues caused by the large amount of WGA lectin in our wheat eating populations is to notice how much glucosamine is sold.

Why? Glucosamine is taken from crustaceans; a large source comes from shrimp. People with joint pain will often take glucosamine to reduce pain and also inflammation. When we take glucosamine, the WGA lectin attaches to it, instead of our tissues. And so we experience less pain or inflammation.

Need more reasons to not eat wheat? There are more. For instance, wheat contains opioid peptides, which may cause an addiction to wheat. And it has been linked to schizophrenia. People with schizophrenia who become gluten-free often see a reduction in their symptoms.

Fast Convenient Foods

Did I mention fast food? No? Let me mention it here. Fast food is generally a GMO product. Meaning the producers fed the animals GMO crops or use GMO crops to make your soy burgers. Frequently, they have raised the animals in filthy, tight quarters that literally drive them insane. These animals are at high risk for disease. They live in agony and are full of terror as they are led to slaughter. Not only is this horrifying to me, but it also releases hormones into the animals' bloodstream. The most noted problems this causes in those that eat the meat are cardiac issues, impotency, and general fatigue.

There is, in general, a lack of nutrients and a high caloric count in the food served by fast food restaurants. The bread is gluten- and sugar-filled. There is also a high amount of chemicals in the food to preserve it and make it taste better. Foods like the ones served at fast food restaurants are what we call empty calorie foods, meaning they have calories, but those calories are void of any value.

Packaged and Convenience Foods from the Grocery Store

Every time another country adopts our eating habits of consuming highly processed foods, their culture becomes more like ours in that they increase their obesity and disease rates.

Packaged and convenience foods from the grocery store are similar to those from fast food restaurants in that they are high in calories, but low in nutritional value.

Here are a few more of the reasons you should not eat them:

- Most processed or packaged foods are high in sugar. I know we already talked about sugar, but let me give you a reminder. Sugar is an empty calorie food. It can lead to the following issues: insulin resistance, high triglycerides, increased cholesterol, increased fat accumulation in the liver, and increased fat accumulation in the abdominal cavity. It is linked to heart disease, diabetes, obesity, and cancer.

- You can actually become addicted to fast foods, craving the dopamine release they give. This leads to overeating and disease.

- Processed foods are high in bad carbs, low in nutritional value, and usually low in fiber.

- These foods are also full of preservatives, added coloring, chemical flavoring, and texturants. These four additives are extremely harmful, and I go over them in more detail in my program, The Healthy Body Program.

Soy

There is so much talk about soy on both sides of the fence. There are people telling you it's healthy to eat and those telling you to avoid it.

The problem is they are both right, as far as eating or not eating it. It's all a matter of how it's produced. If it's fermented (fermenting is important for your health and is covered in the Healthy Body Program), it's safe and healthy to eat. Foods like tempeh, miso, and soy sauce are fermented. Even the Chinese did not eat soy that was not fermented.

Here are some of the reasons you should avoid unfermented soy products:

· **It is toxic.** Unfermented soy contains a lot of natural toxins. These include toxins like enzyme inhibitors, such as trypsin, that prevent protein from digesting. They can cause deficiencies in amino acid and can possibly cause enlargement and other serious conditions of the pancreas, which include cancer.

· **Our bodies react badly to it.** Soy has been shown to cause constipation, sleepiness, and goiters. This has been tested in animals and shown to be true, but I do not believe there has been recorded evidence in humans.

· **It can promote blood clots and the flu.** Unfermented soy has a clot-promoting substance called hemagglutinin, which promotes red blood cells clumping together. It is also found on the surface of influenza viruses and helps them attach to your cells.

· **It depresses the thyroid.** Soy contains goitrogens, which depress the thyroid. If you have thyroid disease, you want to stay far away from non-fermented soy.

- **It harms organs.** About 93 percent of soy is a GMO product. As we know, GMO foods promote cancer and liver and kidney disease.

- **It blocks mineral absorption.** Soy can also block the body's ability to take up essential minerals, such as calcium, iron, copper, magnesium, and zinc. When soy is eaten along with meat, the meat "reduces" the mineral-blocking abilities of the soy. This means meat eaters will still gain some minerals when eating soy but not all that they should gain. It also means that vegetarians who eat soy instead of meat are putting themselves at risk for mineral deficiencies. Animals that are fed a diet of soy must also be fed lysine supplements in order to have normal growth.

When people run out and buy soy burgers, soy milk, edamame (which is what they call soybean eaten as is), dry soybeans, soy nuts, soy sprouts, soy flour, soy cheese(emulating dairy cheese), soy ice cream, they may be thinking they are eating healthy choices, but, in reality, they are harming their health and their family's health.

So what kinds of soy products can you eat? Safe soy foods include natto (a smelly stringy fermented soy food not usually eaten in the U.S.); miso (a fermented soy paste often used in soup and other dishes); tempeh (a fermented, cooked soy product that comes in a rectangle that appears to be grains tightly packed together. It is often used in dishes such as reubens, using the tempeh in place of the meat); tamari (soy sauce made from fermented soy paste); and bean curd (coagulation of soy milk). These foods can improve your health and help fight cancer.

So, we have a lot of "don't eats" in this list. But there are also a lot of foods we should eat in here. The question you may have now is, if you eliminate gluten, red meat, bad sweeteners, bad fats, soy, and fast and convenience foods, how do you replace them without missing all that good stuff?

Well, I find that by replacing the "don't eats" with other wonderful choices, you won't really miss anything at all.

There are some great recipes for gluten-free breads and baked goods. Browse through your local bookstore in the cooking section and look for gluten-free cook books. These have recipes for whole meals that were originally made with some sort of gluten added, but they've remade the recipe to a healthier version.

As far as red meat goes, if you're a meat lover, eat chicken, turkey, duck, or fish. Try more vegetarian meals. Maybe make a day or two every week vegetarian night. Youmay find that you are just as satisfied with the wonderful options that are out there. I'm not talking about frozen soy burgers; I highly recommend that you do not consumethose!

But there are a lot of bean recipes that are filling and full of healthy nutrients. Try veggie dishes with egg for a protein. Or delve into the knowledge that most humans eat too much protein and that there is protein in all veggies. You'll be fine with a veggie dish a few nights a week. In fact, not only will you be fine, but you'll be healthier for it.

Learn how to substitute maple syrup or local honey with white sugar. You can still have healthy sweeteners if you're a sweet tea drinker, you take sugar in your coffee, or you just like a sweet treat now and then.

Bad fats are simply not worth the risk they pose. Use avocado; coconut oil; olive oil; or hormone- and antibiotic-free, pasture-raised, humanely-raised butter. In today's society, it is not hard to find a health food store, and most of them carry all of the above.

Fast and convenience foods, though they save us time and energy, can easily be replaced with healthy, home-cooked or raw foods. With a little planning and preparation, you can easily make simple, fast, healthy meals with fresh ingredients.

And if you have to have soy, you can still eat it–just stick to the healthier, fermented forms.

So where is the list that tells us what we should make sure to add into our diets?

The following is that list. These are foods that fight cancer. If they are organic, they are healthy, flavorful, and full of nutrients:

- Garlic (raw is best)

- Berries (organic)

- Tomatoes (better if slightly cooked)

- Cruciferous vegetables (broccoli, cabbage, cauliflower, brussels sprouts, etc.) (If you have thyroid disease, be sure to only eat cruciferous veggies if they arecooked and limit your amount.)

- Green tea

- Oatmeal and brown rice (in limited amounts)

- Quinoa

- Turmeric

- Leafy green vegetables (Collard greens, mustard greens, kale, romaine lettuce, etc.)

- Grapes (best with seeds)

- Beans (dry beans soaked, not canned)

- Mushrooms (cooked only)

- Onion

- Bone broth

There is an exception to the following list. That would be nightshades. Vegetables in the nightshade family include, but are not limited to, white potatoes, tomatoes, bell peppers, cayenne, chili peppers, habanero, eggplant, goji berries, paprika, and tobacco. There are more, but I believe these are the most common.

Nightshades have an alkaloid called solanine that can cause joint and muscle pain, stiffness, slow healing, arthritis, insomnia, gall bladder issues, heart burn, and/or GERD.

They also contain nicotine, which can make them addictive. (I'll bet you weren't expecting that one.)

Solanine is a poison whose effects can cause gastrointestinal and neurological issues. If you are sensitive to solanine, you may notice that, after eating potatoes or tomatoes, you experience any of the following: nausea, diarrhea, stomach cramps, vomiting, burning in the throat, cardiac dysrhythmia, and/or headache and dizziness. More severe effects include hallucinations, the loss of sensation, jaundice, dilated pupils, fever, paralysis, and/or hypothermia.

Solanine is a defense mechanism that the plant produces naturally to protect itself. If you opt to eat potatoes, never eat them if they are green, especially green under the skin. This means they have been sitting in sunlight and have produced solanine into the danger levels. Potatoes that have sprouts are also extra high in solanine.

The World Health Organization has actually set an upper limit of 20 mg per 100 grams of solanine per the weight of potatoes. They cannot legally be sold in stores if they are above that limit because they are considered too toxic.

Now that you are armed with that information, note that tomatoes are listed in the foods you should eat due to their bountiful health benefits. They are a great source of vitamins A and C and also folic acid. They contain a wonderful variety of nutrients and antioxidants. They have alpha-lipoic acid, lycopene, choline, beta-carotene, potassium, and lutein.

Tomatoes have also been linked to heart health. They have been shown to help lower LDL cholesterol, total cholesterol, and also triglycerides. They also help keep your platelet cells from clumping together. The amount of potassium they have may help lower blood pressure.

Additionally, tomatoes are known to fight free radicals that cause cancer. The lycopene in them is known to fight prostate cancer, so tomatoes can be an important part of a man's diet.

Please just use your own common sense when dealing with tomatoes and other nightshades. If you think you are sensitive to them, you will want to avoid them as much as possible. But if not, they can be a great, healthy addition to your diet.

Chapter 6

In chapter five, we found a lot of information about food and diet. There is a lot to digest in that chapter. You may need to reread it and/or take notes. But there is more that needs to be done to heal the body.

Here, in chapter six, we start by looking at other ways to improve your health and move toward that vision of how you want your life to be.

Meditation is one of the best ways to heal. For one thing, it's free. It's calming, reduces stress, reduces aging, prompts creativity and imagination, helps you feel connected, boosts brain function, helps you feel happier, helps you sleep better, lowers blood pressure, reduces anxiety, reduces headaches, improves joint issues, boosts metabolism and helps aid in weight loss, boosts your immune system, increases your attention span, increases your energy level, improves breathing and heart rate, lowers heart and brain issues, lowers inflammation, lowers asthma attacks, lowers menopause symptoms, also helps prevent arthritis and also fibromyalgia, helps with memory recall, decreases ADHD, increases grey matter in the brain, reduces risk of stroke, helps against Alzheimer's and premature death, improves your relationships and your empathy, decreases feelings of loneliness, and helps with emotional eating.

Dang! There is not a drug on this planet that can do all of that!

If you are new to meditating, don't worry. It's pretty easy to do. There are many ways to meditate.

Here is a simple beginners' way:

Find a quiet place where you won't be distracted. Start with just five minutes a day and work up to a minimum of twenty minutes. After only a couple of weeks of twenty minutes per day, you should start to feel the rewards.

Wear loose and comfortable clothing, and turn off your distractions, like the phone or TV. If you live where you have background noise, try adding your own background whitenoise, like a water fountain, a CD of waves, forest sounds, or chanting meditation music. With practice, you will learn to ignore the outside noises. You should be able to hearthem without letting them distract you from your focus.

Get comfortable, and since you're going to be sitting for a while, it's good to do some stretches first. Then sit comfortably. You'll want to learn to sit in a meditative pose, but for starters, just sit in a way that is comfortable to you. Use good posture.

It's easier for most people to close their eyes, but once you've mastered sitting and focusing, you can leave your eyes gently open if you prefer. Some people like to light acandle and focus on the flame. Others close their eyes and follow their breath.

Let go of your worries and concerns; let go of the list of things you want to complete for the day. If you are wanting to change something in your life, like your health, stateyour intention for your health, "I am healthy; my body is healing; I love my healing body," and repeat it several times until you feel your mind settle down into this belief. Then let that thought go, and simply follow your breath with your mind. Without controlling your breath, follow it into your lungs; watch it swirl around, feeding your body oxygen;then follow it back out into the air; follow into your lungs, and repeat. While you are doing this, you will find thoughts drifting into your mind, distracting you. Simply tell each thought you are aware that it is there and that you'll deal with it later. Send the thought on its way, and follow your breath into your lungs.

If you set a timer, you'll know when you are finished. I like to wait until I "feel" finished. Sometimes I'm surprised at how long I have been meditating. I come out refreshed and full of energy.

There are many other ways to meditate, but this is a simple way to start, and if you practice this every day, you will see benefits.

If you are in my program, you will be doing a guided meditation with me over the phone, and you'll also be receiving a meditation CD in the mail to use at your leisure.

Guided meditation is marvelous and can have powerful effects on the body, right down to the cells. A guided meditation is when you sit and begin to meditate, and someone is there talking you through the meditation. Generally, they are narrating a scene for you to imagine as you listen along. The narrator will help you to relax in mind and body.

Then you are often asked to walk through a field or down a path. You may be asked to meet a guide in your vision or talk to an animal. Sometimes it's a guided tour to visualize your chakras and to heal them. Whatever the narrator is helping you with, he or she will lead you gently through the meditation, helping you to relax and heal.

One of the wonderful things about the mind is that it does not know the difference between reality and imagination. But this can be good and bad, as your brain creates new pathways with each experience you have. This is true whether the event is real or imagined.

On the positive side, during a guided journey by a narrator, the two of you have a goal to work toward in the meditation. The mind can relax and heal. You can change the way your cells are functioning through guided work. And you can even overcome some of life's stressors.

But in the same way, this can be bad when people are stressed out and worried. They imagine the worst thing that could happen and fret over it. Again, the brain does not know that this is imagined worry. It releases the hormones to fit the situation and can cause harm to the body.

That is why taking the time to meditate can be so powerful. While your unfocused mind can often wander to places that can be counterproductive to your health, meditation, on the other hand, can calm the mind and help you heal.

Chapter 7

Now we need to discuss exercise. For many, that is a dreaded topic. People don't want to get off the couch and move. We find we sit all day behind a computer, and when we get home, we want to sit and relax.

The problem with that is it's really unhealthy.

Our bodies are designed to move; we are designed to walk, sprint, bend, stretch, and move in order to survive. Unfortunately today's society has us sitting at a desk to survive. Our social needs have changed, but our physical needs have not.

It isn't that you are lazy. Sitting at work teaches the body to be sedentary. It's like Newton's First Law, "An object at rest stays at rest, and an object in motion stays in motion..." This is true of our bodies as well as any other object. Sitting at work is staying at rest, and when we get home, we want to stay at rest.

In order to stay healthy, we need to move our bodies. Just like Newton's law, we need to get our bodies in motion. Once we switch our mode of thinking over to letting our bodies be in motion, we will want to stay in motion.

I watched an interview with Dick Van Dyke the other day. He is eighty-nine years old and dancing like a forty-year-old. He said he has always exercised. This is a quote from his interview: "In my thirties, I exercised to look good; in my fifties, I exercised to stay fit; in my seventies, I exercised to stay ambulatory; and in my eighties, I exercise to avoid assisted living." And, of course, being as it is Dick Van Dyke, he laughs at the end. He also said he always dances. He is a wonderful example of a body in motion staying in motion.

We all need a little more Dick Van Dyke in us.

If you haven't exercised for a while, you will want to start out easy—taking a walk around the block. If the weather is bad, you can go mall walking. Start out with just ten minutes of movement and build up to an hour a day. An hour goes by quickly if you're being active. Maybe you have a dog; take him for a walk. You'll both benefit from the exercise; you'll bond; and you'll both be in a happier mood when you're done.

I find yoga is one of the best exercises that a person can find. Have you ever taken a good look at singer Adam Levine's muscles and body structure? He says he practices yoga every day, no matter where he is. Some other big names that you might know that practice yoga regularly include Jennifer Aniston; S ting and his wife, Trudie Styler; Jon Bon Jovi; super model Alessandra Ambrosio; Madonna; Gwyneth Paltrow;Jenny McCarthy; Matthew McConaughey; Reese Witherspoon; Robert Downey Jr.; and Woody Harrelson.

WOW, that is a good-looking list. Look these people up if you don't know who they are; they are all easy to find on the Internet. They are all famous, so you'll find a lot of photos of them. Check out their bodies! Every single one of these people practice yoga on a regular basis. There are a lot more people that could be added to that list, but I think you get the idea. Yoga is how these celebrities stay physically and mentally fit. That should be enough of an incentive to at least get you thinking about starting your own yoga practice.

Besides looking good, there is an old saying that says, "You are as young as your spine is flexible, and yoga can do this for you as well. Plus, there are even more reason to get started.

Yoga can...

Improve your flexibility as you bend and stretch your body to the point of strengthening muscles, but not to the point of pain.

Help realign your bones back where they belong.

· Stop cartilage and joints from wearing down. The basic routine moves your joints around in a way that replenishes nutrients in the cartilage.

- Protect the discs in your spine. The discs sit between your vertebrae that make up your spine. As with joint cartilage, your discs need movement to remove the old nutrients stuck inside them, so they can uptake fresh nutrients to stay healthy.

- Improve balance and posture. As you hold positions, you are building muscle strength, which helps with your posture. This can help relieve back and neck pain, and it improves your balance. As you practice, you will find yourself holding your own weight in some poses.

- Strengthen your bones. As you get older, one of the biggest fears is falling and breaking a bone. Yoga lowers your chance of falling and strengthens your bones in case you do fall. This helps your bones get stronger and helps eliminate the threat of osteoporotic fractures.

- Lower the amount of the stress hormone cortisol in your system. This helps you maintain your calcium levels.

- Improve your circulation. As you twist, bend, and move your body, you are forcing your blood to move in and out of organs, and you're also moving blood from your hands and feet more easily. You get more oxygen into your blood this way. Yoga has been shown to create less sticky platelets; this thins the blood and lowers clot-promoting proteins. So you have a lower risk of having a heart attack or stroke.

- Clear out your lymph system. When you bend and twist, you are helping move your lymph system and clearing it out. Your lymph system fights infection and gets rid of toxic waste created by your cells. It helps fight cancer cells!

- Lower your blood pressure and aids in the regulation of your adrenal glands.

- Lower depression, which gives you a happier and more hopeful outlook.

- Lower blood sugar.

- Improve your cholesterol levels by lowering the bad cholesterol and increasing the good.

- Help you focus better on tasks.

- Help your nervous system and relaxes you so you can think clearer and lowers the amount of stress hormones running around in your body.

- Promote better sleep.

- Help prevent illness.

- Strengthen your lungs and you lower your risk of getting digestive issues, including IBS or constipation.

- Remove pain from your body and increase your self-esteem.

- Quiet your mind to help you become calmer and live longer.

I cannot think of a longer and more beneficial list for any other type of exercise. It's not hard to do yoga. You bend as far as you can. That's it. You aren't trying to match the teacher who has, likely, been practicing for years. You are just doing what you are able to do. There is no stress, or demands, on how well you have to do in any pose. You'll get better by daily practice.

And if you buy a CD to follow, or a book, you don't need a membership. You can follow your book or CD free of charge after the initial purchase. In my program, HealthyBody, I send you a gift of a yoga CD and also a yoga mat to practice on.

So there are no excuses. It's not overly strenuous, and you don't need a membership. Practice yoga a little every day and walk every day, and you'll start noticing the difference in a few weeks.

Chapter 8

There is one last thing I'd like to talk about, and that is sleep. Sleep is probably a lot more important than you realize, and seven out of ten Americans are not getting the proper sleep, putting them at risk for serious health issues. In fact, Americans are so sleep-deprived that most of us do not know what it feels like to be fully alert and awake.

New research shows that sleep is a major regulator for your health. Lack of sleep can cause all sorts of physical problems such as:

·   Impaired immune system

·   Inflammation,

·   Damage to your genes

·   Memory loss

·   Slowed reflexes and impaired decision-making skills

·   Hearing loss

·   Impeded sexual function

·   Increased risk of cancer, heart attack, stroke, and insulin resistance and type 2 diabetes

·   Apnea

·   Psychiatric impairments

·   High cholesterol, atherosclerosis, and high blood pressure with a 45 percent higher risk of heart attack

- Headaches

- Vision problems including blurred vision, floppy eyelid syndrome, glaucoma, and temporary blindness

- Increased levels of cortisol, a hormone associated with stress

- Increased food cravings and hunger

- Muscle weakness and decreased athletic performance

- Skin problems and rashes, including eczema

- Hair loss

- Disrupted metabolism, weight gain and obesity

Sleep also affects your long-term memory, emotional stability, cognitive skills, and ability to learn.

And…if you don't get proper sleep after studying, then you won't retain what you learned. It is through sleep that we create our memory. As little as losing an hour a night can affect your learning. There was a study done where adolescents were allowed to come to school an hour later so they could sleep in. The entire school's grade average went up, along with a decrease in flu and colds.

Furthermore, if you are predisposed to a disease, and you don't get adequate sleep, you can bring the disease on fifteen years earlier than it would have shown up; i.e., Alzheimer's at fifty-five instead of seventy.

Now, we have heard a lot of how not getting sleep can be detrimental to your health. The good news is that, when a person restores their body, or trains it, to get proper sleep at night, much of the damage done can be reversed.

Sleep Can Fight Cancer

There is a new study out that shows that how well you sleep can determine how well your body fights cancer. There are three different substances in our bodies that control how well we can avoid or control the growth of cancer in our bodies. They are cortisol, melatonin, and tumor necrosis factor (TNF).

Cortisol is the stress hormone trigger. It increases during times of anxiety and stress, and it is believed that it worsens cancer along with other diseases. Cortisol regulates immune system activity, including the "natural killer" cells that go out and fight cancer. Cortisol levels peak around dawn and decline throughout the day. People that work second shift have cortisol levels that peak in the afternoon. These people typically die earlier from breast cancer. People who wake up a lot during the night also have abnormal cortisol patterns.

Melatonin, a hormone that lowers estrogen production, is produced during sleep. It has antioxidant properties that can help prevent the damage to cells that create cancer.

The cancer killer or tumor necrosis factor is produced in our body at night. People who do not get proper sleep have less and weaker TNF than those who go to bed earlier and sleep through the night.

These three things, though they work in different ways, are very important for preventing and controlling cancer. Getting the right amount of sleep, at the right times, can ensure that they are released in sufficient quantities to control or even prevent cancer.

Other Ways Sleep Improves Health

Besides helping prevent or kill cancer, people who get a proper night's rest find they are happier and healthier. When we sleep, our bodies get busy repairing damage caused during the day. We repair our muscles and bones while we sleep.

Have you ever had a cold, and the doctor told you to drink plenty of fluids and get some rest? There is an actual reason why you are being told to do this. Your body can fight off infections better when you aren't busy doing all those daily activities. You are repairing tissues and muscle cells, which is allowing you to build muscle.

People who get a good night's rest on most nights have healthier skin, are less likely to take risks with their finances, have less need to see the doctor, can pronounce words better, have fewer migraines, and are more focused. They are also generally more productive at their job, have higher libidos and are likely to have better sex, have better vision, and don't make as many dangerous errors. Furthermore, their pain tolerance is higher and their reaction time is better, so they are safer drivers.

In other words, get your rest; it's for your own good

Conclusion

To sum it all up, we have to look at our whole self if we want to heal. We cannot focus only on diet or soul or physical work and expect to be a healthy being.

I know I said this before, but I highly recommend rereading this book and taking notes. Start slow and make the changes in your diet that are stopping you from healing orthat are causing you to become sick.

Write out how you would like to see your life in six months.

Then start walking and learning how to do yoga.

Next add in meditation.

And seek out someone who can help hold you accountable. That makes your work so much easier. We all need to be supported.

This book is my way of supporting you. From the bottom of my heart, I wish you all the health you desire.

About the Author

Cathy Ostema is a holistic health coach, raw food chef, and writer. She has a degree in Social Work, is a Certified Holistic Health Coach, and has helped people in a wide variety of lifestyles, from the mentally and physically ill and/or handicapped, to those with obesity and cancer, to healthy individuals that are looking to increase their love lives or start new careers.

Spending time with family and friends is as important to her as her writing and ability to help others. She happily lives in the Smokey Mountains where she wakes up every day to the call of the healing vortexes. Supported by her husband and family to pursue her life dreams, she spends a lot of her time researching in order to help others heal.

Cathy spent a large portion of her life with a thyroid disease that didn't register on tests by Western medical standards. This led her to begin her own research and find her own cures. Now she is passing that knowledge on to her readers.

www.ingramcontent.com/pod-product-compliance
Lightning Source LLC
Chambersburg PA
CBHW061802280526
45787CB00003BA/1445